Table of Contents

Pollen Count: Understanding and Monitoring Pollen Levels

1. Introduction to Pollen and Pollen Count

To provide patients relief and to prevent the onset of symptoms, many healthcare practitioners review questionnaires and local meteorological data. In order to adapt treatment schedules for individuals living in a given area, it would be of value to have data on the relative abundance and types of exposure for a whole population. This article discusses the technology used in pollen counting and the techniques used to analyze and manually count pollen samples. In addition, the monthly classification of pollen seasons and the diasmic phase are included in the article.

Pollen is a powdery, typically yellow substance that consists of microscopic male reproductive cells in seed plants and is capable of fertilizing the female reproductive cells in the same plant species. It is an essential component of the flowering plants that are required for reproduction. They become more prevalent in the atmosphere of some countries and can influence the incidence and outcome of allergic diseases, which are related to the pollen season start and the daily atmospheric pollen counts. An established and growing area of research is concerned with the measurement of these exogenous factors, which, together with other data, allows medical and industry professionals to develop a better understanding of the prevalence and incidence of allergic diseases in various countries. It has been shown that allergic airways conditions such as asthma and allergic rhinitis are strongly affected by exposure to airborne pollen allergens. Regular monitoring of the levels of pollen in a given region can provide valuable data on levels of exposure to sensitizing allergens for people living in the same area.

2. The Importance of Monitoring Pollen Count

Trees, weeds, and grasses are collectively referred to as 'pollen producers' and their presence in an area results in an obvious increase in medical visits for allergic-related healthcare. People who suffer from allergic diseases-mostly, pollen-related symptoms-such as conjunctivitis, rhinoconjunctivitis, rhinitis, allergic eczema, pollen-food syndromes, and acute urticaria experience severe pollen-related allergic reactions. Allergic symptoms can significantly impact an individual's quality of life and can increase their healthcare costs. Therefore, monitoring and the 'first alert' in the release of pollen levels are essential for trying to avoid or mitigate clinical symptomatology. One possibility of counteracting these issues is to warn and protect individuals from the exposure to pollen triggers.

It is critically important for individuals and government bodies to have a clear understanding of the amount and types of pollen in the atmosphere, which is known as 'pollen count'. Some of the reasons why monitoring pollen count is so important include behavioral composition, health, and medical aspects. For years, the allergic diseases have increased significantly worldwide. In China, as the last national prevalence survey of children and adolescents undertaken from 2010 to 2012, approximately 4-15% of children and 6-23% of adolescents were diagnosed with allergic rhinitis according to a significant variation in the criteria used by the doctors. Allergic people who have a high sensitivity to pollen levels will show several symptoms that can have a strong impact on their day-to-day activities and, in turn, the evening activities during spring. Based on previous studies, during the peak pollen level in spring, over 30% of affected-allergic individuals have severe reactions to pollen.

3. Common Types of Allergenic Pollen

- Oak – pollen from oak trees is likely to cause an allergic reaction, in part because of specific proteins found in their pollen and specific amino acid sequences. These are typically designated as Querc a 1 and/or Querc a 2. - Birch – trees of the Betula genus, commonly known as birch trees, can also cause symptoms. Maples can also fall under this category. The specific protein that can trigger a reaction in someone sensitive is typically categorized as Cor a 1. There is also a sequential homologue (protein with a very similar amino acid sequence) called Cor a 8 found in hazelnuts, a related plant. People allergic to Amb a 1 tend to be affected by this allergen the worst of all and are more likely to develop severe symptoms. - Box Elder (Ash Leaf Maple) – trees of the Acer genus, such as box elder, can cause symptoms. People who are allergic to Birch trees are more likely to be affected by this plant for unknown reasons. - Cedar – species of Juniperus, such as mountain cedar, are well-known for causing allergy symptoms in the winter or early spring, even though many of them have berries. Because pollen from this tree can drift, it causes allergic reactions in people who live far away from it. Sycamore, worked or derived from Acer pseudoplatanus, causes allergy symptoms in some people. It is a sequential homologue to Bet v 1, so a Melchior system would list it as a tango tree. The same may be applicable to other Maples, such as silver or sugar. - Pine – trees of the genus Pinus can also cause symptoms. Individual species can be responsible. Some spruces (Picea) can cause allergy symptoms. Most cedars, worked hybrids, and junipers do not cause allergy symptoms in people. - Grass (Poaceae) Timothy (Cat's Tail) – many of the grasses can cause suffering with the right genetic combination. The most common is allergic reactions to bent, redtop and fescue grasses, but the top of the allergy stack is typically for timothy pollen. Several date varieties must be taken into account in regard to this specific pollen, but a measurement of about 50-60% of the grasses is the most common.

Most tree pollens that are likely to trigger an allergic reaction contain different types of proteins that can cause symptoms. The most common tree pollens that are known to cause these types of issues often have pollen types with these proteins:

4. Tools and Techniques for Pollen Count Measurement

Traditionally, pollen count has been measured using a Burkard volumetric trap. The trapped pollen is then quantified using one of various techniques, such as basic microscopy to count the grain numbers. Other classic methods for pollen count quantification include electronic particle counting based on dispersed light, using a range of laser-based techniques including particle holography, cytometry, holographic microscopy, and dynamic image analysis. In contrast, surrogate techniques such as the Durham sustained release of allergen (Durham SRAT) method and electrostatic rod (Skerman) precipitator use inert solid bodies impregnated with silicone grease to compare the transfer coefficient between a known amount of allergen and the air. Other techniques, such as the volumetric Hirst sampler for non-pollen particulates and the Rotorod sampler for pollen and other bioparticles, are used for background air quality studies. Pollen grain quantity estimates are based on the knowledge of the flow rate of the air through the instrument and of the size or weight of the trapped material. These systems are not valid for estimating the quantity of airborne birch pollen.

The measurement of pollen count or concentration has traditionally been reported as an average value per unit volume of air over between 24 hours and 1 week and is usually expressed as grains per cubic meter of air (grains/m3). Falling under the branch of aerobiology, the field of pollen monitoring takes advantage of a diverse array of instruments and techniques to track, quantify, and forecast pollen levels. Methods for measuring pollen count and pollen concentration fall into one of two classifications: volumetric or surrogate.

5. Local vs. National Pollen Count Data

There are many different ways to monitor the pollen count. The types of pollen monitors include Burkard spore traps, Rotorad Mark II sampler, or a Durham Hirst sampler. This means that the pollen count can be measured in a couple of manners, with one being able to monitor data in real-time and another that can monitor the level of coverage in the environment. A lot of these similarly consist of traps that collect pollen at different intervals of time. Traps can be hand cleaned from time to time and identified and counted under a microscope in order to estimate the amount of pollen in the air. Hand counting is usually conducted using a glass microscope slide upon which the sticky sampling substrate has been collected over a pre-defined sampling interval of time. After removing the slides, they can then be sent to a central analysis facility for counting, which usually takes 5-7 working days to be fully analyzed to produce the pollen count. Pollen counting involves the identification and counting of pollen grains found on a slide or sticky glass plate. These grains are then chemically dissolved and the remaining residue can be further examined for grain types overlooked in the initial assessment. The counting of pollen grains is then used to create a paper or digital graph that shows the levels of different types of pollen for a given area. From this information, it is possible to determine what times of the year different pollens tend to be high.

Airborne Pollen Monitoring

People who experience hay fever or pollen allergies can monitor the pollen count in a number of ways. There are many online resources that can keep you updated with the local state of pollen. This can also provide broader national information that can focus on local areas and give you an indication of the pollen count as well.

6. Factors Affecting Pollen Levels

A national approach to pollen monitoring, in conjunction with traditional signaling systems, is necessary but must also be in accord with this malleable baseline. At the local level, factors will be unique to the particular locality. These locally specific issues must be addressed heuristically by those most familiar with the area. It is often a good idea to list a variety of plants from the area in order to demonstrate the different types of situations that one may need to manage, rather than the spectacular flowers that may be in bloom. It is also a good idea to document particular events such as rainfall, bushfires, high-pressure systems, dust storms, and the like. These can all have profound influences on the local flora. A daily weather log is also useful. With years of data, a small analysis of factors known to increase pollen levels can be undertaken.

A number of factors influence pollen levels on any given day. Among them are factors that humans have control over, such as extensive and predictable urban tree planting, pollution levels, and the absence or presence of environmental management and planning - factors that are inextricably linked. Others are natural or biological phenomena, in a state of great flux from year to year: annual weather patterns (including wind speed and direction), the absence of pathogens and exotic pests, historical planting practices (some exotics can persist for hundreds of years), and frequency, nature, and occurrence of rainfall events. The absence of this mosaic of factors does not allow easy predictions of what types of plants will be in flower at any given time but also makes for floristically interesting cities. Interestingly, as long as urban and peri-urban climate and weather patterns differ, urban vegetation will differ from surrounding native vegetation.

7. Health Impacts of High Pollen Counts

The health risks associated with pollen vary with the concentrations of pollen in the air. Clinical and epidemiological studies have shown that when a hay fever sufferer is exposed to just one pollen grain per cubic metre of air, he or she shows nasal itching, the only symptom of hay fever. When they are exposed to 10 pollen grains per cubic metre of air, he or she shows an increase in nasal itching, running nose and sneezing. At 30 to 50 pollen grains per cubic metre, the eyes start to show symptoms and at higher concentrations of 50 to 100 pollen per cubic meter, severe hay fever symptoms are exhibited. Based on these studies, the Met Office forecasts for pollen types are offered as a scale of nil, low, moderate, high or very high. Although, it is typical for 10 to 15% of any population to show symptoms of hay fever, over this percentage could suffer when pollen count is high.

Day-to-day exposure to pollen can affect health. High pollen levels affect a large proportion of the population, those with hay fever and/or asthma which, in the UK, could mean more than 15 million people. When these individuals are exposed to high pollen counts, either daily over the pollen season or following sudden peaks in pollen levels, their hay fever symptoms can be heightened. They are also more likely to require medication, to report more severe hay fever, and they are more likely to have an asthma attack. It is not just people with these conditions who are affected; when pollen levels are high, even those who do not usually suffer allergy symptoms may develop hay fever and/or asthma. Furthermore, high pollen levels have been shown to directly affect symptoms and lung function among patients with chronic obstructive pulmonary disease, and pollen spores can exacerbate the adverse effects of exposure to man-made pollution.

8. Strategies for Managing Allergy Symptoms

Knowing when allergenic pollen counts will be high or low is helpful. This can help people predict which parts of the year will tax their immune systems, and allow them to take steps to "pre-inflammatory". If the body doesn't start with a high immune system load, there will be some burden it can handle when more is gradually added, instead of becoming suddenly full. Check the internet for automated updates on the level of pollen for your location. A large number of sites track allergenic pollen for different localities every day, sometimes every few hours, and report an allergy index that rates the occurrence of allergens for that day as being very low, low, moderate, high, or very high. Many city health departments maintain allergen websites and send assistance reports during adverse weather conditions. Filters for heating, ventilation, and air conditioning units in cars, homes, and offices can help to reduce the amount of pollen inhaled when turned on, and keep the air inside the building cleaner. They can also be combined with personal breathing zone filters in especially allergenic conditions. Since high quality whole-house HVAC filtration is typically seen as an absence of infestation, however, it may not be the best solution for allergic asthma, where small amounts of pollen can be intensely irritating.

Involuntary pollen exposure becomes a major problem for several groups of people every time of the year. Pollen allergies manifest symptoms characteristic of respiratory pathologies, skin abnormalities, and the alteration of the ocular surface of the eye. Although pharmacological treatments associated with pollen exposure are mainly used, the combination with avoidance strategies, especially when pollen exposure is associated with high allergen concentrations, provides effective symptom relief. Persons with recent pollen allergies and a diagnosis of asthma are most at risk for experiencing allergies or asthma due to the characteristics of the allergens. There are eight robust strategies to alleviate allergies. Some are preventative (you stop the symptoms before the pollen arrives); others are restorative (you treat the symptoms after they appear). These can be applied in an elementary fashion by the individual. Some of these may seem odd or unusual, but remember: because allergies are the result of a pollen-triggered hyper-reactions immune system, methods to relieve or terminate symptoms might be different from the familiar methods for treating a standard cold or influenza. These diverse methods for relief and treatment are based upon either side of the three pathways outlined above. Some serve to avoid the arrival of the allergens, and the rest work to negate the hyper-reactions brought about by the allergens.

9. Incorporating Pollen Count into Daily Routine

There are a number of options: here are a few. Semi-automated solutions include the following. Whenever you read your physical or virtual newspaper, watch the weather forecast on TV, or log onto a website such as the World Meteorological Organisation or a national meteorological service site, also access the pollen count if it is available. View or set up an RSS or Atom feed for your chosen weather website if it has one. Use the feed reader utility to monitor the feed and to give you a list of weather, including the pollen count, whenever any new weather is available. Vacation planner. Either set up hacks or register with an alert service that will email you the pollen count on the eve of outdoor events such as a family day out.

If pollen causes a problem for you, then why not automatically build a check for the pollen count into your daily routine? Not only that, but why not automatically build knowledge or hacker scripts to interact with this component of the world when the pollen count is released in a format and location that you can use? Keep in mind that the pollen count often changes from day to day.

10. Innovations in Pollen Count Tracking Technology

Technology is being researched to develop an AllergyTrigger based on the commercial sensor that is able to accept this treatment. Additionally, an air filter inside a home could lower indoor pollen counts. It would be important for those who suffer from allergies to know when a filter is working well and an inexpensive real-time pollen monitor would allow just that. Overall, the combination of open data, miniaturized low-cost electronic sensors, and machine learning tools to process air quality data has the potential to greatly expand our understanding of where and when people are at risk for exposure to unhealthy environmental conditions. As we advance in technological development and these delightfully shrinking particle swarms start to influence more and more weather and climate models, we may see a more direct impact of this tech on disaster preparedness and public health in the future.

A promising tool in tracking and sensing of pollen is being deployed in different spaces. In tracking solids in the space available for a single pollen grain, electrostatic, as well as optical, tools have proven to be useful. Particles, such as air pollutants, that are roughly the same size as pollen are already being tracked by a number of commercial and academic entities at the urban scale. The most recent step in technology is to create a real-time pollen tracking sensor for the average consumer.

With global warming and climate change around us, tracking is now even more important than ever. With citizens and professionals now tracking pollen count, reports to remove affected plants from a lawn will only be somewhat helpful now. Urban planners and biologists, too, are studying pollen counts to decide where to place trees that produce less pollen. Engineers are interested in counting seed hairs in the air to better predict bird strikes when airplanes take off or land.

Understanding Pollen Allergies: A Comprehensive Guide

1. Introduction to Pollen Allergies

One in five individuals in the United States reports having been diagnosed with allergies, including allergic rhinitis, eczema, asthma, and other allergic reactions. Allergic diseases, including allergic asthma, are on the rise, posing severe social and economic difficulties, but the reasons are poorly understood. Rhinoconjunctivitis or seasonal allergic rhinitis is the most common, being prevalent globally. One of the major sources of causative agents of nasal allergic rhinitis is from tree and grass pollens. While for some individuals, it may clear within a span of a few days, but in 40% of the affected population, allergic rhinitis symptoms last for several weeks and can progress to have a negative impact on the quality of life as chronic rhinitis. Factors that impact the severity and impacts on rhinitis will be discussed here. It is generally well accepted that the allergens found in these grains are the most common sources of allergic reactions to pollen. However, allergic rhinitis and asthma can be provoked by certain fruits and vegetables that can cross-react with pollen in individuals who are already allergic.

"What doesn't kill you makes you stronger." While in certain contexts, this statement might hold true, but not when it comes to pollen allergies. In practice, it is one of the leading causes of chronic illnesses in the United States. It provokes an allergic response when certain airborne pollen grains, primarily the grains from wind-pollinated plants, are inhaled. A sudden surge of exposure often causes symptoms of pollen allergy to become increasingly problematic, particularly in people who live in urban settings where lack of fresh air and open spaces intensify the uncontrolled environmental pollen exposure. Furthermore, climate change has led to an extended pollen season and higher pollen load in the environment, causing a great impact on health worldwide. In this feature article, we have reviewed the different approaches and treatment strategies currently in practice for decreasing the progression and/or controlling the symptoms related to pollen allergies to improve the quality and standard of life of the sufferers.

2. Types of Pollen Allergies

Weed allergy: Ragweed is the primary cause for allergies in the autumn. Native to the US, it now grows in many parts of the world, including Europe and North America. A single ragweed plant, according to the Asthma and Allergy Foundation of America, may produce up to one million particles of pollen into the atmosphere. The pollen was discovered upwards into the atmosphere as high as a mile and a half. Most allergic reactions in humans result from inhaling airborne pollen.

Grass allergy: Common all over the world, grass allergy is particularly prevalent in the United States. Signs of a grass pollen allergy may appear between late spring and early summer, peaking at the end of June. Timothy, Bermuda, and Johnson grasses are the three major types of grasses that have an effect on seasonal allergies. Individuals with a grass allergy may also be allergic to certain plants, such as tomatoes, watermelons, oranges, and peaches. In late spring and early summer, tree pollen allergies are at their peak. People with allergies to one type of tree may also experience reactions to other varieties of tree pollen. The following are some of the most frequent tree pollen allergies: Oak, Alder, Birch, Cedar, Elm, Maple, Ash, Cottonwood, Pine, Poplar.

When discussing pollen allergies, it's important to keep in mind that there are different sources of pollen. Different plants and trees produce pollen at different times, potentially causing symptoms to span the entire year.

2.1. Grass Pollen Allergy

This means grass pollen allergy can be widespread, and pollen can be found in most outdoor places. Grasses are of most concern all over Australia. In most areas, grasses usually flower in the summer months. Single grass species, however, can flower at other times of the year. The grass species that present the greatest allergy problems are recognizable by their feathery or silky flowers. People with grass allergies should avoid mowing lawns and should not allow grass to go to seed around homes. Pets can bring in enough grass pollen on their fur to trigger symptoms in sensitive people. Grass pollen is microscopic and can trigger allergic symptoms even indoors. Stretching membrane air filters are sometimes recommended to remove pollen from indoor air. Optimal long-term management of grass pollen allergy will depend on allergies identified in tests, symptoms, and whether asthma is present. Proper diagnosis by a health professional trained in allergic illnesses is essential to develop an allergy plan.

Grass pollen allergy is a reaction to the pollen released from flowering tops of grasses. This is a very common pollen allergy, often causing hay fever nationwide. In season, pollen from grass is most commonly found in the air. Symptoms of sensitivity to common grass pollen include sneezing, runny or blocked nose, itchy and watery eyes, scratchy or sore throat, shortness of breath, and wheezing. Other symptoms include fatigue and irritability.

Pollen from grass can be transported by the wind for hundreds of kilometers and is well-distributed.

2.2. Tree Pollen Allergy

Tree pollen allergy symptoms vary, but often resemble hay fever. Individuals may experience sneezing, itchy, watery eyes, a runny or stuffed nose, and/or cough. Additionally, some may experience headaches, impaired sense of smell, or pandas. Chronic conditions that may seem unrelated to the sinuses or lungs may also worsen with a pollen allergy. Upper airway symptoms typically occur when pollen comes into direct contact with the sinuses. More rarely, the allergens may embed in mucus faster than the body breaks them down, resulting in symptoms similar to food allergy, food intolerance, or acid reflux. The sensation can also lead to the "globus" of "lump in the throat" feeling. Itchiness may present as a "brain itch," an unusual but not painful sensation. In fact, an itchy mouth or throat without hives is the most common food allergy "reaction" in people with OAS/PFS.

· Allergenic tree species, especially in certain regions, include acacia, ash, aspen, beech, birch, box elder, cedar, cottonwood, date palm, elm, hickory, juniper, larch, locust, maple, mountain cedar, mulberry, oak, olive, palm, pecan, pine, poplar, redwood, sycamore, walnut, western red cedar, and willow. · When trees produce "catkin" flowers, they too may be a source of allergenic pollen. · As with all allergens, the amount of pollen in the air can vary, and pollen levels may also be affected by weather conditions or local air quality. Dry, windy weather often leads to higher pollen levels, but clip art showing leaves on trees, and even swollen buds, may be misinterpreted as "high pollen" conditions. Disturbances in swollen buds, such as through grooming or petting, can sometimes release an even larger burst of pollen than a warm, sunny, dry day. · Some people have both a fresh and a tree-pollen-food allergy. These are often referred to as Oral Allergy Syndrome (OAS) or Pollen-Food Syndrome (PFS). This means that when someone eats a fresh version of a fruit, they have tingling, itching, or even a swollen or itchy throat and possibly other symptoms; but they do not have the same reaction from cooked versions of the foods they are allergic to. Typically, larger trees with airborne pollen are involved in these reactions, but not poplar.

2.3. Weed Pollen Allergy

Simple mask carriers used to protect against large particle inhalation in allergen avoidance studies have resulted in a 52-81% reduction in allergen-induced nasal obstruction in weed-allergic patients. Allergen avoidance methods studied for hay fever include wearing a mask during the season, using filters on heating, air conditioning, and windows, irrigation or washing away pollen from the eyes, nasal passages, and airways, applying topical nasal corticosteroids and antihistamines with minimal systemic effects are all used in managing symptoms of weed pollen allergy. For example, budesonide (Rhinocort Aqua), triamcinolone (Nasacort), mometasone furoate (Nasonex), fluticasone (Flonase). Desensitization methods for weed pollen allergy include sublingual immunotherapy (SLIT), or administering low doses of allergen to increase tolerance, along with injection immunotherapy.

Control and Management

Allergic symptoms triggered by weed pollen exposure tend to appear in susceptible individuals who are exposed, although intermediate responses may be detected utilizing allergy skin tests. In addition to the classic nasal and ocular symptoms of hay fever, other organ systems can be involved in sensitized individuals. These include bronchial asthma from seasonal allergy to pollen allergens and contact dermatitis to herbal products. These complaints are not so easily related to pollen sensitivity because hay fever symptoms are characteristic. Manifestations on the skin include acute allergic contact dermatitis with multiple, very pruritic, flat erythematous raised wheals (urticaria); allergic contact dermatitis; and other pruritic skin eruptions on the face, neck, chest, back, and arms caused by exposure to plant pollen surrogates/extracts.

Allergic Symptoms

Species of ragweed, the Composite Family and Amaranth family elicit many allergic symptoms. Common weeds associated with pollen allergies include nettle, ragweed, parietaria, plantain, pellitory/butterweed/futh, cocklebur, wormwood or wormseed/mugwort, our lady's keys, eyebright, daisy, and goldenrods. Other weeds of relatively minor importance are burning bush, Christmas rose, bursage/buckwheat tree, poverty weed, firebush, camel thorn, chaparral, ironwood, beat Ginger, spleenwart, kasandra, bur sage, and icaco.

3. Symptoms of Pollen Allergies

Asthma is a reversible obstruction of the airways due to bronchospasm from inflammation, increased mucus, and swelling of the airways. The major symptom is shortness of breath from wheezing and coughing. Treatment and prevention consist of avoiding known allergens, medications to stabilize the immune system, reduced inhalant exposure, and symptom management. Whether they are airborne or carried by other methods, allergens commonly cause hay fever. More than 25% of Americans are affected by hay fever. In Western countries, greater than 50% of the population is sensitized to one or more allergens. In the United States, total exposure to pollen may range from 10,000 to 30,000 grains of pollen/m3 of air.

Sneezing is a common complaint during the pollen season. One may also feel like clearing his or her throat or coughing following a sneeze. The nose runs, causing itching of the nose and postnasal drip, resulting in clearing of the throat, cough, and sore throat. The nose may be more stopped up or congested, decreased in smell, and at times, lead to sinus infections (sinusitis). The ears also may feel stopped up. Allergic shiners (black eyes) are a result of swelling and discoloration from venous congestion from chronic backflow from the nose. Fatigue is a common symptom. Although rare, some individuals may experience shortness of breath due to asthma. Decreased performance may be a consequence of poor sleep or sleep apnea. Whites of the eyes may become red and may have difficulty wearing contact lenses. Direct contact with pollen can cause inflammation of the eyelids and conjunctivitis, which can occur throughout the year.

4. Diagnosis and Testing for Pollen Allergies

The healthcare professional may conduct a skin prick test by pricking, puncturing, or cutting the skin and applying a dilution of an allergen. The results can be read roughly 15–20 minutes later by examining the extent of redness and swelling at the site. If the patient experiences allergies, the test is positive, with larger wheals ("welts") typically indicating a greater sensitivity to the allergen. Healthcare professionals can also perform an intradermal (skin) test to diagnose a patient with suspected indoor allergies (e.g., to cat, dog, dust mites) whose skin prick test results are negative or indeterminate. Intradermal testing is chosen based on the presence of clinical symptoms after significant animal exposure (e.g., dog groomers, pet store employees) and can result in false positives in feed stores with significant environmental air exposure. Healthcare professionals can draw blood from a patient to measure the quantity of specific IgE antibodies that are attacking a foreign substance that enters the body, also known as allergens or antigens. A normal result indicates no sensitization, reactivity, allergy, or untoward effect to specific allergens tested. If the anti-IgE result indicates a positive reaction, then the patient is considered sensitized or reactive to the specific allergen or allergens tested.

The tests that healthcare professionals may use to diagnose pollen allergies are physical examinations, detailed accounts of the patient's symptoms and health history, as well as measurement of IgE antibodies via skin or blood tests. Allergists are trained to recognize the triggers that are causing your current symptoms by asking careful, detailed questions about what happens before, during, or after symptoms appear as well as inquiring about the anatomy and practices related to your home, work, and hobbies. In addition to a person's history of symptoms, treatments, family history, and exposure to allergens, physical examinations and available technologies (e.g., stethoscope, tongue depressor, nasal speculum, light source, spirometry) are used by allergists to differentiate between causes of symptoms and plan treatment and management accordingly.

Diagnosis and Testing

5. Treatment Options for Pollen Allergies

Immunotherapy is a treatment option for patients over 5 years of age suffering from seasonal allergic diseases. Immunotherapy is a disease modifying treatment that treats the underlying cause of your allergies. We offer allergy immunotherapy in the form of Allergy Drops. The goal of immunotherapy is to modify the body's response to offending allergens, thus inducing allergen-specific tolerance and decreasing the allergic symptoms produced upon natural exposure to the allergen. There are two main ways that the allergy shots/drops work to decrease one's allergy symptoms. The first is by changing the immune system, telling the allergy system to turn off and stop reacting against the allergens it once reacted significantly against. The second means by which allergy shots/drops may improve symptoms is by the natural degradation of allergic antibodies over time. With regular and consistent dosing over time, the amount of the allergic antibody (IgE) in the system may decrease.

There are several treatment options for pollen allergies, ranging from over-the-counter (OTC) medications to allergy immunotherapy treatment offered by board-certified allergists like those found at the Allergy & Environmental Treatment Center, LLC. OTC medications include decongestants, antihistamines, steroids, cromolyn sodium, or a combination of antihistamines and decongestants with or without pain relievers. The most potent common OTC medications are antihistamines, which can also help treat other symptoms of allergic rhinitis, such as itching, hives, and allergic conjunctivitis. Taking an antihistamine will help to neutralize histamine levels, reducing itching and tearing caused by naturally released histamine. Some other helpful medications are those designed to treat a cough. In addition, eye drops, nasal sprays, oral decongestants, oral antihistamine, or common pain killers may be used, along with acetaminophen if alternative pain relieving medications are not recommended or not effective at reducing a headache.

5.1. Medications

Make an appointment with your GP or a specialist if you are suffering signs of severe allergies, including those affecting your daily life, avoiding activities, being less productive at work or school, or being unable to sleep. A variety of alternative care plans are available to those who are unable to use drugs due to health conditions or are seeking to explore other options. In these situations, OTC medications (including antihistamines and decongestants) can still be productive, as well as some prescription medications such as intranasal antihistamines and corticosteroids. Furthermore, targeted immunotherapy is a preventative therapy that can suppress allergies for a long time, lasting for at least 3 to 4 years. However, not every person is able to begin oral immunotherapy, and not everyone is able to see a separation of drugs. To find a care strategy that works adequately, make an appointment with your doctor.

Antihistamines block the release of histamine by a type of immune cell known as the mast cell, thus decreasing or preventing symptoms. Decongestants make swollen nasal tissue shrink and bring the underlying blood vessels back to their normal size. They work by narrowing the blood vessels, which decreases the flow of blood. As a result, the swelling shrinks, and the tissues no longer feel stuffy. However, it is important not to take decongestants for longer than a week at a time because this can lead to a rebound effect. Regular use of decongestants can also interfere with sleep. Antihistamines and decongestants are often combined into a single pill. For example, patients can use cetirizine for allergies due to pollen and a combination of fexofenadine and pseudoephedrine when an oral decongestant is indicated. Nasal steroids reduce inflammation in the nasal passages and are considered the best therapy for allergies in the nose. They work by reducing the body's ability to secrete antibodies after exposure to allergens. Nasal DNAase, intranasal antimuscarinics, and intranasal antihistamines are newer medications that have been approved for use in persistent or severe symptoms. These medications can be used in addition to, or in some cases, instead of nasal corticosteroids. Two of these medications are described here.

Over-the-counter (OTC) and prescription medications can help with symptoms and, in some cases, help with the underlying mechanisms that cause these symptoms. Your doctor will help you decide which medications you need and how to take them according to your allergies.

5.2. Immunotherapy

Individuals may have the option of observing reactions at a healthcare facility. Most patients will develop a tolerance for their allergens, resulting in a gradual decrease in the frequency of healthcare provider visits. According to the Asthma and Allergy Foundation of America (AAFA), up to 85 percent of individuals who receive immunotherapy experience substantial symptom relief. Conversely, sublingual immunotherapy might be used to treat allergies, but the most common is to use allergy tablets. These are the same as the shots, but instead of symptoms, the allergen is held under the tongue for 30 seconds and then swallowed. The American College of Allergy, Asthma, and Immunology has developed sublingual drops that are placed under the tongue. They also provide symptom reduction, but the effects might wane rapidly if therapy is not continued. This technique is not yet widely used, and further research is required to establish its long-term efficacy. With both shots and tablets, the allergist/immunologist must have prior knowledge and experience with the method.

Immunotherapy may be considered as a long-term strategy for treating pollen allergies. In the case of allergy shots, an individual is typically administered a dosage containing a small amount of the allergen, which is gradually increased over time. This treatment option can help desensitize the body and reduce or prevent allergic reactions. The approach takes time to work; an allergic individual might require regular shots for numerous months or years.

According to the American Academy of Allergy, Asthma & Immunology (AAAAI), allergy shots are an effective method of reducing or preventing allergy symptoms for many individuals. Allergy shots are typically given about once a week or as frequently as once a month. After reaching the maintenance stage, shots are usually given every four weeks and may be administered for an additional three to five years to enhance results.

6. Prevention and Management Strategies

• Lifestyle Adjustments - Products that can cause pollen to spread and trigger symptoms, such as hair dryers, candles, perfumes, commercial cleaning products, air fresheners, and window fans, should be avoided. Low-maintenance plants, as well as a small number of organic candles, air purifiers, or a growing number of company products that have achieved the Asthma and Allergy Foundation of America's (AAFA) Allergy Control Certification, can also be highlighted. Allergen-proof pillow, mattress, and box spring encasements can also help individuals reduce their allergen exposure.

• Environmental Controls - Homes, school classrooms, and office spaces can be equipped with central air conditioning systems, dehumidifiers, and high-efficiency particulate air (HEPA) filters. These items can trap pollen, preventing it from entering the space and exacerbating allergic symptoms.

• Pollen Avoidance - Recommended during days with high pollen levels and in the morning when exposure is highest. Skipping outdoor activities as well as sporting events can also be useful, just as people can wait until the evening to go outside if possible. Wearing long sleeves, gloves, and sunglasses when outdoors can also aid in preventing pollen exposure. Additionally, air conditioning systems can be utilized while driving or when spending time outside to minimize pollen exposure.

A. Individuals with pollen allergies often employ a variety of methods to reduce pollen exposure and alleviate symptoms. Understanding practical avoidance and environmental control strategies for pollen is the first step in managing pollen allergy symptoms. The following management and changes in the environment or style of life can be achieved.

7. Pollen Count and Forecasting

The present study reports a novel application for finding and predicting the vertical transportation of pollen. ECMWF allows researchers to explore even more vertical information about the atmosphere up to 96 hours in advance of a forecast. It is handy to understand the source of high pollen concentrations and total/vertical loading related to allergenic pollen, as well as to validate the data. Early warning and the spread of pollen grain knowledge are also becoming more important to promote public health. This is the first study to emphasize the ECMWF model as a tool in managing health problems, such as secondary asthma caused by airborne pollen grains growing near urban areas. Pollen grains are often transported by wind and can cause serious symptoms in people who have an allergic reaction when inhaled. Pollen grains are typically released from flowering plants and grasses and then become airborne.

The study assessed the potential of the European Centre for Medium-Range Weather Forecasts (ECMWF) using the European Space Agency (ESA) Climate Change Initiative (CCI) reanalysis product, which includes emissions from the Copernicus Atmosphere Monitoring Service (CAMS) model.

The transition of plant-related emissions and vertical turbulence, coupled with the detection of plant pollen from geostationary satellites, presents new opportunities for pollen sink studies. However, pre-launch validation and

observational gaps make it difficult to exploit these
opportunities.

7.1. Importance of Pollen Count

High pollen counts typically make outdoor conditions unwelcoming for individuals with seasonal allergies. People with pollen allergies can stay indoors during times of high pollen concentration unless essential. When going outdoors cannot be avoided, individuals can take precautions such as using allergy medication or wearing a mask that filters out pollen, as stated by the American College of Allergy, Asthma & Immunology.

Pollen count information helps individuals anticipate possible symptoms related to pollen allergies. Pollen counts are usually aired in weather reports together with weather forecasts. With this information, individuals can make educated decisions such as when to play or walk outside, the right time to start and discontinue certain allergy medications, and what safety measures to take, if any.

Measuring a standard volume of air over a set amount of time can give a pollen count, which indicates how many grains of pollen have been detected. This count is typically reported as grains per cubic meter of air. If a pollen is not reported as having been detected in a sample at a specific time, this indicates that amounts were present in lower amounts than the level of detection for that particular pollen grain (usually around 3 grains per cubic meter of air). Count levels are described by concentrations as none, low, moderate, high, and very high.

Pollen Count

7.2. How Pollen Count is Measured

The size of the area covered might vary depending on the total number of samples already being analyzed and the accuracy and the resources available to project the levels for the area; 2) choose pollen types that will serve as a good index for the most frequent allergenic pollinosis in that area (e.g. Pollen Monitoring Services in the UK have chosen tree pollen levels as a useful index of the likelihood of high allergenic pollen which is more location specific). Chosen pollen types must be identified to species, and be clearly recognizable in the sample. Keep the laboratory's focus on the chosen pollen types to prevent work overload. Measurement of these chosen pollen types does not in any way prevent other pollen types from being reported. It is of course good practice to also report on these other pollen types, which could also be indicators of lesser allergic reactions in sensitized people. In order to be helpful for forecasting services that produce the daily allergy trigger advice, an analysis day should be sufficiently in advance of the forecast day to give a ~ 30 h delay for staining, and a minimum of 4 h for counting the slides.

Pollen meteorology investigates the state of pollen in the atmosphere, and the amount and composition of biological particles is expressed as pollen count. There are several ways to assess the pollen count in the environment. Pollen count is determined by taking into account the number of pollen grains of anemophilous plants qualitatively and quantitatively in the samples collected from the air. The techniques developed for measurement of allergenic pollen count, sampling, microscopy and data analysis, are helpful in assessing the level of risk for people allergic to the pollen of anemophilous plants on that respective day. This work presents the standard guidelines for measuring the level and concentrations of the pollen count.

7.3. Tools for Tracking Pollen Count

Using open-source forecasting data such as weather sensors and machine learning, companies and organizations that track and predict pollen count like these may have already prepared a platform that people are already interacting with. The National Allergy Bureau (NAB) (U.S.) has a mobile app and a website where anyone can check their local pollen count. Users of the AirVisual Air Quality App can use the application or visit IQAir.com. The European Aeroallergen Network (EAN) through Eurac Research's Allergy Diary app, Byosystems today, Pollenguru, other pollen diary applications, and the Copernicus Atmosphere Monitoring Service (CAMS) also use this information for their pollen forecasts and archives.

Since keeping track of local pollen count is essential to manage pollen allergies, people can access forecasts from various sources. Allergen tracker apps, these applications, typically free and available in app stores like Apple Store and Google Play, allow users to monitor the prediction and occurrence of different types of pollen throughout the year to better treat their allergies. Smart devices, personal computers, and tablets are compatible with these software. Websites from third parties such as The Weather Channel, Pollen.com, and Accuweather allow users to check reliable and localized pollen forecasts to help them prepare for allergies. Many of these websites, as well as the apps mentioned above, provide reports on allergy flares and air quality in addition to pollen forecasts.

8. Impact of Climate Change on Pollen Allergies

These changes in environmental parameters can affect all stages of the pollen cycle. For example, trees and weeds of the same species can have both a longer pollen flow and a greater pollen production. Several studies have shown the influence of CO2, inseparable from climate change, on pollen production and allergenic potential, demonstrating increased production in the roots of the plant, in the flower, in the fruits, and in the pollen that is thrown. Regarding the reproductive phase, different authors refer to a trend towards greater allergenic potential if the pollen is produced around 700 mbar, which will facilitate the diffusion of the pollen that affects us so much. There is predictive evidence that both seasons and the allergic impact of the pollen produced by these trees are changing. These findings do not yet allow us to know if this change is due to greater biological fluidity or if it also implies the loss of these pollens or their allergenic capacity.

The world is changing faster and faster every year, and the environment is no exception. The increase in greenhouse gases, pollution, or massive deforestation are just some of the examples of the way humans are altering the environment. Another major impact is climate change, and with it, the increase in the prevalence and sometimes the aggressiveness of pollen allergies.

9. Common Misconceptions about Pollen Allergies

3. Myth: The pollen count is only important if you have specific allergies to certain types of pollen. Pollen from trees, grasses, and weeds are the most significant allergy triggers nationally. The pollen count measures the amount of pollen, known as pollen surface grains, in a cubic meter of air in a given area at a specific time. Mold spores are also counted as part of the pollen count. Under ideal weather conditions, pollen measures are taken daily to determine how much pollen is in the air and what type(s) of pollen are causing you issues. While the pollen count may help you confirm that pollen exposure is the current source of your allergic symptoms, you can still have an allergy to pollen even when the "numbers" are "low."

2. Myth: Pollen allergies only occur in those who have had symptoms during their childhood. You can develop allergies at any age, including pollen allergies. Allergies can come and go in some people. Peak onset is usually in adolescence.

1. Myth: People with asthma also have pollen allergies. Pollen allergies can trigger asthma. Asthma induced by pollen is commonly known as "allergic asthma."

Here are nine common misconceptions.

Pollen allergies are often misunderstood. Dispelling some of the most common myths surrounding the condition could help you get an accurate diagnosis, find effective treatment, and give you the knowledge you need to manage your symptoms and condition.

10. Resources for Individuals with Pollen Allergies

Visiting a Healthcare Provider That Can Help: - Ear, nose, and throat doctors (otolaryngologists) may also be able to diagnose and treat allergic rhinitis. Many ear, nose, and throat doctors specialize in treating diseases of the ear, nose, and throat, but some have also received additional training in the treatment of allergies as well. - Nurse practitioners, physician assistants, or other healthcare providers can also diagnose and provide tailored treatments for allergic rhinitis/pollen allergies. Many of these healthcare providers have also received additional training in the treatment of allergies, including the diagnosis and treatment of allergic rhinitis/pollen allergies.

Educational Materials: - Brochures in English and Spanish on allergic rhinitis (hay fever) and asthma related to hay fever are available from the American Academy of Allergy, Asthma, and Immunology. They may be ordered from their website. - Patient advocacy organizations may also have educational materials available on allergic rhinitis, hay fever, and asthma related to allergic rhinitis. Examples include: - Allergy and Asthma Foundation of America - Asthma and Allergy Network - Books on allergic rhinitis/hay fever may also be available at a local library or bookstore.

Other Online Forums: - The American Academy of Allergy, Asthma, and Immunology offers an online forum for patients to seek out reliable news related to allergies/immunology. - MedHelp offers forums on allergies that are actively monitored by healthcare workers/social workers who can often answer questions. - There are many online chat forums where individuals with food allergies can chat, interact, seek advice, and/or support. However, the information posted on these sites is opinion, not fact-based. That being said, the information and support may be beneficial for some individuals. Some of the food allergy forums are hosted on websites such as: - PeanutAllergy.com - KidsWithFoodAllergies.org

- Many patient advocacy organizations offer support for individuals with allergic rhinitis, hay fever, and/or asthma. Many of them offer support groups and chat sites/forums for patients to interact with one another, ask questions, seek advice, and/or support one another. Examples include: - Asthma and Allergy Foundation of America - Allergy and Asthma Network - American Partnership for Eosinophilic Diseases - Food Allergy Research and Education

Patient Advocacy Organizations: